The Complete Lean & Green Lunch Cookbook

Delicious Lean & Green Lunch Recipes For Beginners

Jesse Cohen

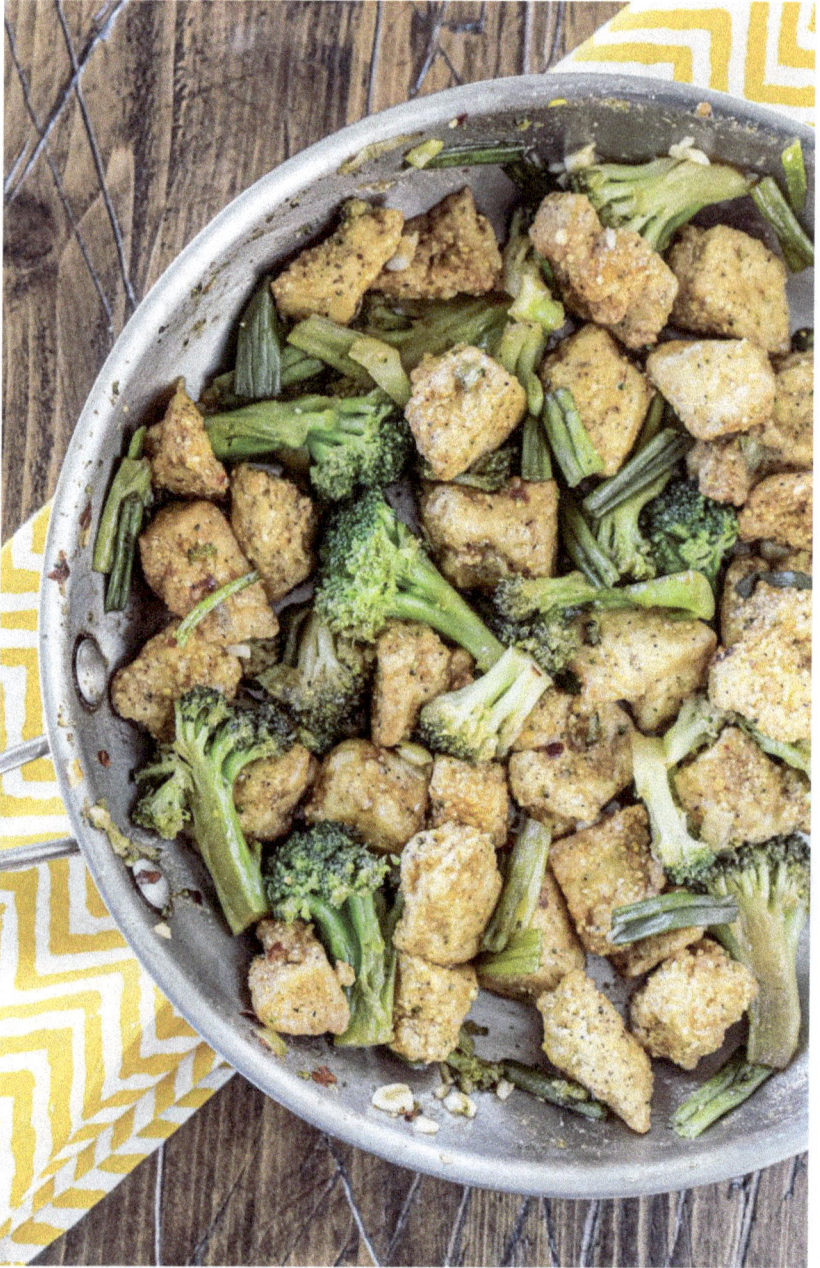

Table of contents

Tofu with Broccoli

Servings: 4

Preparation Time: 20 minutes

Cooking Time: 25 minutes

Ingredients:

For Tofu:

- 14 ounces of firm tofu, drained, pressed and cut into 1-inch slices
- 1/3 cup of arrowroot starch, divided
- ¼ cup of olive oil
- 1 teaspoon of fresh ginger, grated
- 1 medium onion, sliced thinly
- 3 tablespoons of low-sodium soy sauce
- 2 tablespoons of balsamic vinegar
- 1 tablespoon of maple syrup
- ½ cup of water

For Steamed Broccoli:

- 2 cups of broccoli florets

Instructions:

1. In a shallow bowl, place ¼ cup of the arrowroot starch.
2. Add the tofu cubes and coat with arrowroot starch.
3. In a cast-iron wok, heat the vegetable oil over medium heat and cook the tofu cubes for about 8-10 minutes or until golden from all sides.
4. With a slotted spoon, transfer the tofu cubes onto a plate. Set aside.
5. In the same wok, add ginger and sauté for about 1 minute.
6. Add the onions and sauté for about 2-3 minutes.
7. Add the soy sauce, vinegar and syrup and bring to a mild simmer.
8. In the meantime, in a small bowl, dissolve the remaining arrowroot starch in water.
9. Slowly, add the arrowroot starch mixture into the sauce, stirring continuously.
10. Stir in the cooked tofu and cook for about 1 minute.
11. Meanwhile, in a large pan of water, arrange a steamer basket and bring to a boil.
12. Adjust the heat to medium-low.
13. Place the broccoli florets in the steamer basket and steam, covered for about 5-6 minutes.
14. Remove from the heat and drain the broccoli completely.
15. Transfer the broccoli into the wok of tofu and stir to mix.
16. Serve hot.

Tofu with Peas

Servings: 5

Preparation Time: 15 minutes

Cooking Time: 20 minutes

Ingredients:

- 2 tablespoons of olive oil, divided
- 1 (16-ounce of) package extra-firm tofu, drained, pressed and cubed
- 1 cup of yellow onion, chopped
- 1 tablespoon of fresh ginger, minced
- 2 garlic cloves, minced
- 1 tomato, chopped finely
- 2 cups of frozen peas, thawed
- ¼ cup of water
- 2 tablespoons of fresh cilantro, chopped

Instructions:

1. In a non-stick wok, heat 1 tablespoon of the oil over medium-high heat and cook the tofu for about 4-5 minutes or until brown completely, stirring occasionally.
2. Transfer the tofu into a bowl.

3. In the same wok, heat the remaining oil over medium heat and sauté the onion for about 3-4 minutes.

4. Add the ginger and garlic and sauté for about 1 minute.

5. Add the tomatoes and cook for about 4-5 minutes, crushing with the rear of a spoon.

6. Stir in the peas and broth and cook for about 2-3 minutes.

7. Stir in the tofu and cook for about 1-2 minutes.

8. Serve hot with the garnishing of cilantro.

Tofu with Brussels Sprout

Servings: 3

Preparation Time: 15 minutes

Cooking Time: 15 minutes

Ingredients:

- 1½ tablespoons of olive oil, divided
- 8 ounces of extra-firm tofu, drained, pressed and cut into slices
- 2 garlic cloves, chopped
- 1/3 cup of pecans, toasted and chopped
- 1 tablespoon of unsweetened applesauce
- ¼ cup of fresh cilantro, chopped
- ½ pound Brussels sprouts, trimmed and cut into wide ribbons
- ¾ pound mixed bell peppers, seeded and sliced

Instructions:

1. In a skillet, heat ½ tablespoon of the oil over medium heat and sauté the tofu for about 6-7 minutes or until golden brown.
2. Add the garlic and pecans and sauté for about 1 minute.

3. Add the applesauce and cook for about 2 minutes.

4. Stir in the cilantro and take away from heat.

5. Transfer tofu into a plate and put aside

6. In the same skillet, heat the remaining oil over medium-high heat and cook the Brussels sprouts and bell peppers for about 5 minutes.

7. Stir in the tofu and take away from the heat.

8. Serve immediately.

Tofu with Veggies

Servings: 4

Preparation Time: 20 minutes

Cooking Time: 45 minutes

Ingredients:

- 1 (14-ounce of) package extra-firm tofu, pressed, drained and cut into small cubes
- 2 tablespoons of sesame oil, divided
- 4 tablespoons of low-sodium soy sauce
- 3 tablespoons of maple syrup
- 2 tablespoons of peanut butter
- 2 tablespoons of fresh lime juice
- 1-2 teaspoons of chili garlic sauce
- 1-pound green beans, trimmed
- 2-3 small red bell peppers, seeded and cubed
- 2 scallion greens, chopped

Instructions:

1. Preheat your oven to 400 degrees F.
2. Line a baking sheet with parchment paper.

3. Arrange the tofu cubes onto the prepared baking sheet in a single layer.

4. Bake for about 25-30 minutes.

5. Meanwhile, in a small bowl, add 1 tablespoon of the olive oil, soy sauce, maple syrup, spread, lemon juice, and chili aioli and beat until well combined. Set aside.

6. Remove from the oven and place the tofu cubes into the bowl of sauce.

7. Stir the mixture well and put aside for about 10 minutes, stirring occasionally.

8. With a slotted spoon, remove the tofu cubes from the bowl, reserving the sauce.

9. Heat a large cast-iron skillet over medium heat and cook the tofu cubes for about 5 minutes, stirring occasionally.

10. With a slotted spoon, transfer the tofu cubes onto a plate. Set aside.

11. In the same skillet, add the remaining vegetable oil, green beans, bell peppers and 2-3 tablespoons of reserved sauce and cook, covered for about 4-5 minutes.

12. Adjust the heat to medium-high, and stir in the cooked tofu remaining reserved sauce.

13. Cook for about 1-2 minutes, stirring frequently.

14. Stir in the scallion greens and serve hot.

Tofu & Mushroom Curry

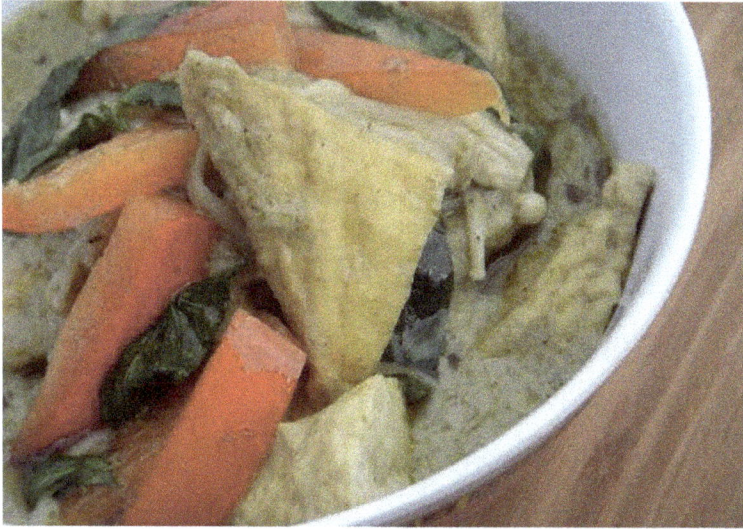

Servings: 4

Preparation Time: 20 minutes

Cooking Time: 25 minutes

Ingredients:

For Tofu:

- 16 ounces of extra-firm tofu, pressed, drained and cut into ½-inch cubes
- 1 garlic clove, minced
- 3 tablespoons of balsamic vinegar

- 3 tablespoons of low-sodium soy sauce
- 3 tablespoons of arrowroot starch
- 2 tablespoons of sesame oil
- 1 tablespoon of Erythritol
- 1 teaspoon of red pepper flakes
- 2 tablespoons of coconut oil

For Curry:

- ¼ cup of water
- 1 small yellow onion, minced
- 3 large garlic cloves, minced
- 1 teaspoon of fresh ginger, grated
- 2 cups of fresh mushrooms, sliced
- 3 tablespoons of red curry paste
- 13 ounces of light coconut milk
- 1 tablespoon of low-sodium soy sauce
- 2 tablespoons of fresh lime juice
- 1 teaspoon of lime zest, grated
- 8 fresh basil leaves, chopped

Instructions:

1. For tofu: in a resealable bag, place all ingredients.
2. Seal the bag and shake to coat well.
3. Refrigerate to marinate for 2-4 hours.

4. In a large skillet, melt the coconut oil over medium heat and fry the tofu cubes for about 4-5 minutes or until golden brown completely.
5. With a slotted spoon, transfer the tofu cubes into a bowl.
6. For curry: in a large pan, add the water over medium heat and bring to a simmer.
7. Add the minced onion, garlic and ginger and cook for about 5 minutes.
8. Add the mushrooms and curry paste and stir to mix well.
9. Stir in the remaining ingredients apart from basil and simmer for about 10 minutes.
10. Stir in the tofu and simmer for about 5 minutes.
11. Garnish with basil and serve.

Tofu & Veggies Curry

Servings: 5

Preparation Time: 20 minutes

Cooking Time: 30 minutes

Ingredients:

- 1 (16-ounce of) block firm tofu, drained, pressed and cut into ½-inch cubes
- 2 tablespoons of coconut oil
- 1 medium yellow onion, chopped
- 1½ tablespoons of fresh ginger, minced
- 2 garlic cloves, minced
- 1 tablespoon of curry powder
- Salt and ground black pepper, as required
- 1 cup of fresh mushrooms, sliced
- 1 cup of carrots, peeled and sliced
- 1 (14-ounce of) can unsweeten low-fat coconut milk
- ½ cup of low-sodium vegetable broth
- 2 teaspoons of Erythritol
- 10 ounces of cauliflower florets
- 1 tablespoon of fresh lime juice
- ¼ cup of fresh basil leaves, sliced thinly

Instructions:

1. In a Dutch oven, heat the oil over medium heat and sauté the onion, ginger and garlic for about 5 minutes.

2. Stir in the curry powder, salt and black pepper and cook for about 2 minutes, stirring occasionally.

3. Add the mushrooms and carrot and cook for about 4-5 minutes.

4. Stir in the coconut milk, broth and sugar and bring to a boil.

5. Add the tofu and cauliflower and simmer for about 12-15 minutes, stirring occasionally.

6. Stir in the juice and take away from the heat.

7. Serve hot.

Tempeh with Bell Peppers

Servings: 3

Preparation Time: 15 minutes

Cooking Time: 15 minutes

Ingredients:

- 2 tablespoons of balsamic vinegar
- 2 tablespoons of low-sodium soy sauce
- 2 tablespoons of tomato sauce
- 1 teaspoon of maple syrup
- ½ teaspoon of garlic powder
- 1/8 teaspoon of red pepper flakes, crushed
- 1 tablespoon of vegetable oil
- 8 ounces of tempeh, cut into cubes
- 1 medium onion, chopped
- 2 large green bell peppers, seeded and chopped

Instructions:

1. In a small bowl, add the vinegar, soy sauce, spaghetti sauce, maple syrup, garlic powder and red pepper flakes and beat until well combined. Put aside.

2. Heat 1 tablespoon of oil in a large skillet over medium heat and cook the tempeh about 2-3 minutes per side.

3. Add the onion and bell peppers and heat for about 2-3 minutes.

4. Stir in the sauce mixture and cook for about 3-5 minutes, stirring frequently.

5. Serve hot.

Tempeh with Brussel Sprout & Kale

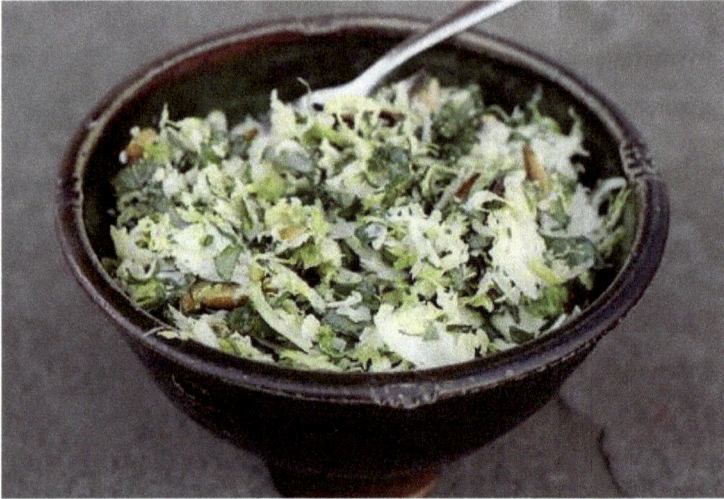

Servings: 3

Preparation Time: 15 minutes

Cooking Time: 17 minutes

Ingredients:

- 2 tablespoons of olive oil
- 1/3 cup of red onion, chopped finely
- 1½ cups of tempeh, cubed
- 2 cups of Brussels sprout, quartered
- 2 garlic cloves, minced
- ½ teaspoon of ground cumin

- ½ teaspoon of garlic powder
- Salt and ground black pepper, to taste
- 2 cups of fresh kale, tough ribs removed and chopped

Instructions:

1. Heat the oil in a skillet over medium-high heat and sauté the onion for about 4-5 minutes.
2. Add in remaining ingredients apart from kale and cook for about 6-7 minutes, stirring occasionally.
3. Add kale and cook for about 5 minutes, stirring twice.
4. Serve hot.

Tempeh with Veggies

Servings: 3

Preparation Time: 15 minutes

Cooking Time: 17 minutes

Ingredients:

For Sauce:

- 3 tablespoons of tahini
- 2 tablespoons of low-sodium soy sauce
- 1 tablespoon of sesame oil
- 1 tablespoon of chili garlic sauce
- 1 tablespoon of maple syrup

For tempeh & Veggies:

- 3 tablespoons of olive oil, divided
- 8 ounces of tempeh, cut into 1x2-inch rectangular strips
- 8 ounces of fresh button mushrooms, sliced thinly
- 8 ounces of fresh spinach
- 1 tablespoon of fresh ginger, minced
- 1 tablespoon of garlic, minced

Instructions:

1. For sauce: in a bowl, add all ingredients and beat until well combined.
2. In a large skillet, heat the oil over medium-high heat and cook the tempeh for about 4-5 minutes or until browned.
3. With a slotted spoon, transfer the tempeh into a bowl and put aside.
4. In the same skillet, heat the remaining oil over medium-high heat and cook the mushrooms for about 6-7 minutes, stirring frequently.
5. With a slotted spoon, transfer the mushrooms into a bowl and put aside.
6. In the same skillet, add the spinach, ginger and garlic and cook for about 2-3 minutes.
7. Stir in the cooked tempeh, mushrooms and sauce and cook for about 1-2 minutes, stirring continuously.
8. Serve hot.

Parmesan Eggs in Avocado Cup

Servings: 2

Preparation Time: 10 minutes

Cooking Time: 12 minutes

Ingredients:

- 1 avocado, halved and pitted
- Salt and ground black pepper, as required
- 2 eggs
- 1 tablespoon of low-fat Parmesan cheese, shredded

Instructions:

1. Arrange a greased square piece of foil in the air fry basket.
2. Select "Bake" of Breville Smart Air Fryer Oven and adjust the temperature to 390 degrees F.
3. Set the timer for 12 minutes and press "Start/Stop" to start preheating.
4. Meanwhile, carefully scoop out about 2 teaspoons of flesh from each avocado half.
5. Crack 1 egg in each avocado half and sprinkle with salt, black pepper and cheese.

6. When the unit beeps to point out that it's preheated, arrange the avocado halves into the prepared air fry basket and insert in the oven.

7. When the cooking time is completed, transfer the avocado halves onto serving plates.

8. Top with Parmesan and serve.

Baked Eggs

Servings: 4

Preparation Time: 10 minutes

Cooking Time: 12 minutes

Ingredients:

- 1 cup of marinara sauce, divided
- 1 tablespoon of capers, drained and divided
- 8 eggs
- ¼ cup of whipping cream, divided
- ¼ cup of low-fat Parmesan cheese, shredded and divided
- Salt and ground black pepper, as required
- 4 cups of fresh baby spinach

Instructions:

1. Grease 4 ramekins. Set aside.
2. Divide the marinara sauce in the bottom of every prepared ramekin evenly and top with capers.
3. Carefully crack 2 eggs over marinara sauce into each ramekin and top with cream, followed by the Parmesan cheese.
4. Sprinkle each ramekin with salt and black pepper.

5. Select "Bake" of Breville Smart Air Fryer Oven and adjust the temperature to 400 degrees F.

6. Set the timer for 12 minutes and press "Start/Stop" to start preheating.

7. When the unit beeps to point out that it's preheated, arrange the ramekins over the wire rack.

8. When the cooking time is completed, remove the ramekins from the oven.

9. Serve warm alongside the spinach.

Spinach & Tomato Bites

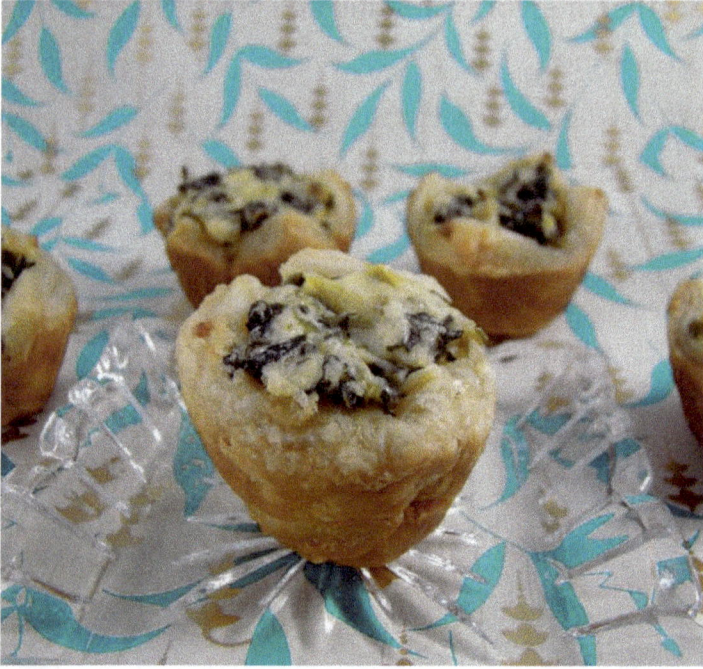

Servings: 2

Preparation Time: 10 minutes

Cooking Time: 30 minutes

Ingredients:

- 4 eggs
- 1/3 cup of spinach, chopped
- ½ cup of tomatoes, chopped

- ½ cup of unsweetened almond milk
- 1 cup of low-fat Gouda cheese, shredded
- Salt, as required

Instructions:

1. In a large ramekin, add all the ingredients and blend well.
2. Place the ramekins in the air fry basket.
3. Select "Air Fry" of Breville Smart Air Fryer Oven and adjust the temperature to 340 degrees F.
4. Set the timer for 30 minutes and press "Start/Stop" to start preheating.
5. When the unit beeps to point out that it's preheated, insert the air fry basket in the oven.
6. When the cooking time is completed, remove the air fry basket from the oven.
7. Serve hot.

Zucchini Omelet

Servings: 2

Preparation Time: 15 minutes

Cooking Time: 18 minutes

Ingredients:

- 1 teaspoon of olive oil
- 1 zucchini, julienned
- 4 eggs
- ¼ teaspoon of fresh basil, chopped
- ¼ teaspoon of red pepper flakes, crushed
- Salt and ground black pepper, as required

Instructions:

1. In a skillet, heat the oil over medium heat and cook the zucchini for about 4-5 minutes.
2. Remove from the heat and put aside to chill slightly.
3. Meanwhile, in a bowl, add the eggs, basil, red pepper flakes, salt and black pepper and beat until well combined.
4. In a baking dish, place the zucchini mixture.
5. Top with egg mixture and gently stir to mix.

6. Select "Air Fry" of Breville Smart Air Fryer Oven and adjust the temperature to 355 degrees F.

7. Set the timer for 10 minutes and press "Start/Stop" to start preheating.

8. When the unit beeps to point out that it's preheated, arrange the baking dish over the wire rack.

9. When the cooking time is completed, remove the baking dish from oven and transfer the omelette onto a plate.

10. Cut into equal-sized wedges and serve hot.

Bell Pepper Omelet

Servings: 2

Preparation Time: 10 minutes

Cooking Time: 10 minutes

Ingredients:

- 1 teaspoon of coconut oil
- 1 small onion, sliced
- ½ of green bell pepper, seeded and chopped
- 4 eggs
- ¼ teaspoon of unsweetened almond milk
- Salt and ground black pepper, as required
- ¼ cup of low-fat Cheddar cheese, grated

Instructions:

1. In a skillet, melt the coconut oil over medium heat and cook the onion and bell pepper for about 4-5 minutes.
2. Remove the skillet from heat and put aside to chill slightly.
3. Meanwhile, in a bowl, add the eggs, milk, salt and black pepper and beat well.
4. Add the cooked onion mixture and gently stir to mix.
5. Place the bell pepper mixture into a little baking dish.

6. Select "Air Fry" of Breville Smart Air Fryer Oven and adjust the temperature to 355 degrees F.

7. Set the timer for 10 minutes and press "Start/Stop" to start preheating.

8. When the unit beeps to point out that it's preheated, arrange the baking dish over the wire rack.

9. When the cooking time is completed, remove the baking dish from oven and place onto a wire rack to chill for about 5 minutes before serving.

10. Cut the omelets into 2 portions and serve hot.

Bell Pepper & Broccoli Omelet

Servings: 4

Preparation Time: 10 minutes

Cooking Time: 2 hours

Ingredients:

- 6 eggs
- ½ cup of unsweetened almond milk
- 1/8 teaspoon of red chili powder
- 1/8 teaspoon of garlic powder
- Salt and ground black pepper, as required
- 1 medium red bell pepper, seeded and sliced thinly
- 1 cup of small broccoli florets
- 1 small yellow onion, chopped
- 2 tablespoons of fresh parsley, chopped

Instructions:

1. In a bowl, add the eggs, milk, chili powder, garlic powder, salt and black pepper and beat until well combined.
2. In a baking dish, mix the bell pepper, broccoli and onion.
3. Pour the egg mixture on top and gently stir to mix.
4. Arrange the baking dish over the wire rack.

5. Select "Slow Cooker" of Breville Smart Air Fryer Oven and assail "High".

6. Set the timer for 1½-2 hours and press "Start/Stop" to start cooking.

7. When the cooking time is completed, remove the baking dish from the oven and transfer the omelets onto a serving plate.

8. Cut into 4 equal-sized wedges and serve hot with the garnishing of parsley.

Mixed Veggie Omelet

Servings: 6

Preparation Time: 15 minutes

Cooking Time: 2 hours 13 minutes

Ingredients:

- 1 tablespoon of olive oil
- 1 medium onion, chopped
- ¾ cup of carrot, peeled and chopped
- ¾ cup of zucchini, chopped
- ¼ cup of green bell pepper, seeded and chopped
- ¼ cup of red bell pepper, seeded and chopped
- ½ cup of low-fat Parmesan cheese, grated
- 8 eggs
- Salt and ground black pepper, as required

Instructions:

1. In a skillet, heat the oil over medium heat and cook the onion for about 2-3 minutes.
2. Add the remaining vegetables and cook for about 8-10 minutes.
3. Remove from the heat and put aside to chill slightly.

4. Meanwhile, in a bowl, add cheese, eggs and black pepper and beat until well combined.
5. In a baking dish, place the vegetable mixture.
6. Pour the egg mixture on top evenly.
7. Arrange the baking dish over the wire rack.
8. Select "Slow Cooker" of Breville Smart Air Fryer Oven and assail "High".
9. Set the timer for two hours and press "Start/Stop" to start cooking.
10. When the cooking time is completed, remove the baking dish from the oven and transfer the omelets onto a serving plate.
11. Cut into equal-sized wedges and serve hot.

Chicken & Bell Pepper Omelet

Servings: 5

Preparation Time: 15 minutes

Cooking Time: 2¾ minutes

Ingredients:

- ½ cup of unsweetened almond milk
- 6 eggs
- 1 garlic clove, minced
- Salt and ground black pepper, as required
- ¾ cup of cooked chicken, chopped
- 1 red bell pepper, seeded and sliced thinly
- 1 small white onion, chopped finely
- 1 cup of part-skim mozzarella cheese, shredded

Instructions:

1. In a bowl, add the milk, eggs, garlic, salt and black pepper and beat until well combined.
2. In a greased baking dish, place the egg mixture.
3. Add the chicken, bell pepper and onion and stir to mix.
4. Arrange the baking dish over the wire rack.

5. Select "Slow Cooker" of Breville Smart Air Fryer Oven and assail "High".

6. Set the timer for 2¾ hours and press "Start/Stop" to start cooking.

7. After 2½ hours, sprinkle the omelets with cheese evenly.

8. When the cooking time is completed, remove the baking dish from the oven and transfer the omelets onto a serving plate.

9. Cut into 4 equal-sized wedges and serve hot.

Turkey & Zucchini Omelet

Servings: 6

Preparation Time: 15 minutes

Cooking Time: 35 minutes

Ingredients:

- 8 eggs
- ½ cup of unsweetened almond milk
- 1/8 teaspoon of red pepper flakes, crushed
- Salt and ground black pepper, as required
- 1 cup of cooked turkey meat, chopped
- 1 cup of low-fat Monterrey Jack cheese, shredded
- ½ cup of fresh scallion, chopped
- ¾ cup of zucchini, chopped

Instructions:

1. In a bowl, add the eggs, almond milk, salt and black pepper and beat well.
2. Add the remaining ingredients and stir to mix.
3. Place the mixture into a greased baking dish.
4. Select "Bake" of Breville Smart Air Fryer Oven and adjust the temperature to 315 degrees F.

5. Set the timer for 35 minutes and press "Start/Stop" to start preheating.
6. When the unit beeps to point out that it's preheated, arrange the baking dish over the wire rack.
7. When the cooking time is completed, remove the baking dish from the oven and place onto a wire rack to chill for about 5 minutes before serving.
8. Cut into equal-sized wedges and serve.

Spinach & Tofu Omelet

Servings: 2

Preparation Time: 15 minutes

Cooking Time: 10 minutes

Ingredients:

- 1 teaspoon of arrowroot starch
- 2 teaspoons of water
- 3 eggs
- 2 teaspoons of red boat fish sauce
- 1 teaspoon of olive oil
- Ground black pepper, as required
- ¼ cup of fresh spinach, chopped finely
- 6 ounces of silken tofu, pressed and sliced

Instructions:

1. In a large bowl, dissolve arrowroot starch in water.
2. Add the eggs, fish sauce, oil and black pepper and beat well.
3. Add the spinach and stir to mix.
4. Place tofu in the bottom of a greased baking dish and top with the egg mixture.

5. Select "Air Fry" of Breville Smart Air Fryer Oven and adjust the temperature to 390 degrees F.

6. Set the timer for 10 minutes and press "Start/Stop" to start preheating.

7. When the unit beeps to point out that it's preheated, arrange the baking dish over the wire rack.

8. When the cooking time is completed, remove the baking dish from oven and place onto a wire rack to chill for about 5 minutes before serving.

9. Cut into equal-sized wedges and serve.

Mini Veggie Frittatas

Servings: 2

Preparation Time: 15 minutes

Cooking Time: 17 minutes

Ingredients:

- 1 tablespoon of coconut oil
- ½ of white onion sliced thinly
- 1 cup of fresh mushrooms, sliced thinly
- 1¼ cups of fresh spinach, chopped
- 3 eggs
- ½ teaspoon of fresh rosemary, chopped
- Salt and ground black pepper, as required
- 3 tablespoons of low-fat Parmesan cheese, shredded

Instructions:

1. In a frying pan, melt coconut oil over medium heat and cook the onion and mushroom for about 3 minutes.
2. Add the spinach and cook for about 2-3 minutes.
3. Remove the frying pan from heat and put aside to chill slightly.

4. Meanwhile, in a small bowl, add the eggs, rosemary, salt and black pepper and beat well.

5. Divide the beaten eggs into 2 greased ramekins evenly and top with the veggie mixture, followed by the cheese.

6. Select "Air Fry" of Breville Smart Air Fryer Oven and adjust the temperature to 330 degrees F.

7. Set the timer for 12 minutes and press "Start/Stop" to start preheating.

8. When the unit beeps to point out that it's preheated, place the ramekins over the air rack.

9. When the cooking time is completed, remove the ramekins from oven and place onto a wire rack for about 5 minutes before serving.

Spinach & Tomato Frittata

Servings: 6

Preparation Time: 15 minutes

Cooking Time: 30 minutes

Ingredients:

- 10 large eggs
- Salt and ground black pepper, as required
- 1 (5-ounce of) bag baby spinach
- 2 cups of grape tomatoes, halved
- 4 scallions, sliced thinly
- 8 ounces of feta cheese, crumbled
- 3 tablespoons of hot olive oil

Instructions:

1. In a bowl, place the eggs, salt and black pepper and beat well.
2. Add the spinach, tomatoes, scallions and feta cheese and gently stir to mix.
3. Spread the oil in a baking dish and top with the spinach mixture.

4. Select "Bake" of Breville Smart Air Fryer Oven and adjust the temperature to 350 degrees F.
5. Set the timer for 30 minutes and press "Start/Stop" to start preheating.
6. When the unit beeps to point out that it's preheated, arrange the baking dish over the wire rack.
7. When the cooking time is completed, remove the baking dish from oven and place onto a wire rack to chill for about 5 minutes before serving.
8. Cut into equal-sized wedges and serve.

Chicken & Veggies Frittata

Servings: 8

Preparation Time: 15 minutes

Cooking Time: 3 hours

Ingredients:

- 8 eggs
- ½ teaspoon of dried parsley
- Pinch of garlic powder
- Salt and ground black pepper, as required
- 1 1/3 cups of cooked chicken, chopped finely
- 1½ cups of red bell pepper, seeded and chopped
- ¾ cup of frozen chopped spinach, thawed and squeezed
- ¼ cup of yellow onion, chopped

Instructions:

1. In a bowl, add the eggs, parsley, garlic powder, salt and black pepper and beat well.
2. In a greased baking dish, place the remaining ingredients.
3. Pour the egg mixture over chicken mixture and gently stir to mix.
4. Arrange the baking dish over the wire rack.

5. Select "Slow Cooker" of Breville Smart Air Fryer Oven and assail "Low".

6. Set the timer for 3 hours and press "Start/Stop" to start cooking.

7. When the cooking time is completed, remove the baking dish from the oven and transfer the frittata onto a serving plate.

8. Cut into 4 equal-sized wedges and serve hot.

Beef & Scallion Frittata

Servings: 4

Preparation Time: 15 minutes

Cooking Time: 20 minutes

Ingredients:

- ½ pound cooked ground beef, grease removed
- 1 cup of low-fat Colby Jack cheese, shredded
- 8 eggs, beaten lightly
- 4 scallions, chopped
- 1/8 teaspoon of red pepper flakes, crushed
- Salt and ground black pepper, as required

Instructions:

1. In a bowl, add the meat, cheese, eggs, scallion and cayenne and blend until well combined.
2. Place the mixture into a greased baking dish.
3. Select "Air Fry" of Breville Smart Air Fryer Oven and adjust the temperature to 360 degrees F.
4. Set the timer for 20 minutes and press "Start/Stop" to start preheating.

5. When the unit beeps to point out that it's preheated, arrange the baking dish over the wire rack.

6. When the cooking time is completed, remove the baking dish from oven and place onto a wire rack to chill for about 5 minutes before serving.

7. Cut into 4 wedges and serve.

Beef & Veggie Frittata

Servings: 2

Preparation Time: 15 minutes

Cooking Time: 14 minutes

Ingredients:

- 1 tablespoon of olive oil
- ¼ cup of cooked ground beef
- 4 cherry tomatoes, halved
- 6 fresh mushrooms, sliced
- Salt and ground black pepper, as required
- 3 eggs
- 1 tablespoon of fresh parsley, chopped
- ½ cup of low-fat Parmesan cheese, grated

Instructions:

1. In a baking dish, place the bacon, tomatoes, mushrooms, salt, and black pepper and blend well.
2. Place the baking dish in the air fry basket.
3. Select "Air Fry" of Breville Smart Air Fryer Oven and adjust the temperature to 320 degrees F.

4. Set the timer for 14 minutes and press "Start/Stop" to start preheating.
5. When the unit beeps to point out that it's preheated, insert the air fry basket in the oven.
6. Meanwhile, in a bowl, add the eggs and beat well.
7. Add the parsley and cheese and blend well.
8. After 6 minutes of cooking, top the bacon mixture with egg mixture evenly.
9. When the cooking time is completed, remove the air fry basket from the oven and transfer the frittata onto a plate.
10. Cut into equal-sized wedges and serve hot.

Pork & Spinach Frittata

Servings: 2

Preparation Time: 15 minutes

Cooking Time: 13 minutes

Ingredients:

- ¼ cup of cooked pork, chopped
- ½ tomato, cubed
- ¼ cup of fresh baby spinach
- 3 eggs
- Salt and ground black pepper, as required
- ¼ cup of low-fat Parmesan cheese, grated

Instructions:

1. In a skillet, heat the oil over medium heat, cook the pork and tomato and cook for about 5 minutes.
2. Add the spinach and cook for about 1-2 minutes.
3. Remove from the heat and put aside to chill slightly.
4. Meanwhile, in a small bowl, add the eggs, salt and black pepper and beat well.
5. In a baking dish, place the pork mixture and top with egg mixture.

6. Select "Air Fry" of Breville Smart Air Fryer Oven and adjust the temperature to 355 degrees F.

7. Set the timer for 8 minutes and press "Start/Stop" to start preheating.

8. When the unit beeps to point out that it's preheated, arrange the baking dish over the wire rack.

9. When the cooking time is completed, remove the baking dish from oven and transfer the frittata onto a platter.

10. Cut into equal-sized wedges and serve hot.

Trout Frittata

Servings: 4

Preparation Time: 15 minutes

Cooking Time: 25 minutes

Ingredients:

- 1 tablespoon of olive oil
- 1 onion, sliced
- 6 eggs
- ½ tablespoon of horseradish sauce
- 2 tablespoons of crème Fraiche
- 2 hot-smoked trout fillets, chopped
- ¼ cup of fresh dill, chopped

Instructions:

1. In a skillet, heat the oil over medium heat and cook the onion for about 4-5 minutes.
2. Remove from the heat and put aside.
3. Meanwhile, in a bowl, add the eggs, sauce Albert, and crème Fraiche and blend well.
4. In the bottom of a baking dish, place the cooked onion and top with the egg mixture, followed by trout.

5. Select "Air Fry" of Breville Smart Air Fryer Oven and adjust the temperature to 320 degrees F.

6. Set the timer for 20 minutes and press "Start/Stop" to start preheating.

7. When the unit beeps to point out that it's preheated, arrange the baking dish over the wire rack.

8. When the cooking time is completed, remove the baking dish from oven and place onto a wire rack to chill for about 5 minutes before serving.

9. Cut into equal-sized wedges and serve with the garnishing of dill.

Tomato Quiche

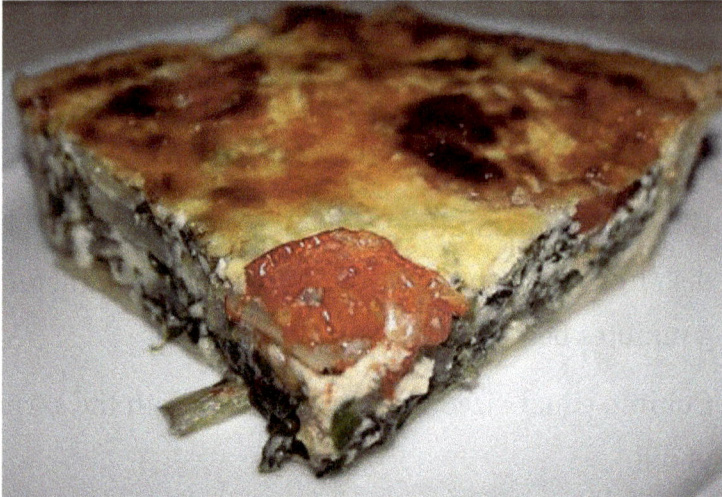

Servings: 2

Preparation Time: 15 minutes

Cooking Time: 30 minutes

Ingredients:

- 4 eggs
- ¼ cup of onion, chopped
- ½ cup of tomatoes, chopped
- ½ cup of unsweetened almond milk
- 1 cup of low-fat Gouda cheese, shredded
- Salt, as required

Instructions:

1. In a small baking dish, add all the ingredients and blend well.

2. Select "Air Fry" of Breville Smart Air Fryer Oven and adjust the temperature to 340 degrees F.

3. Set the timer for 30 minutes and press "Start/Stop" to start preheating.

4. When the unit beeps to point out that it's preheated, arrange the baking dish over the wire rack.

5. When the cooking time is completed, remove the baking dish from oven and place onto a wire rack to chill for about 5 minutes before serving.

6. Cut into equal-sized wedges and serve.

Spinach Quiche

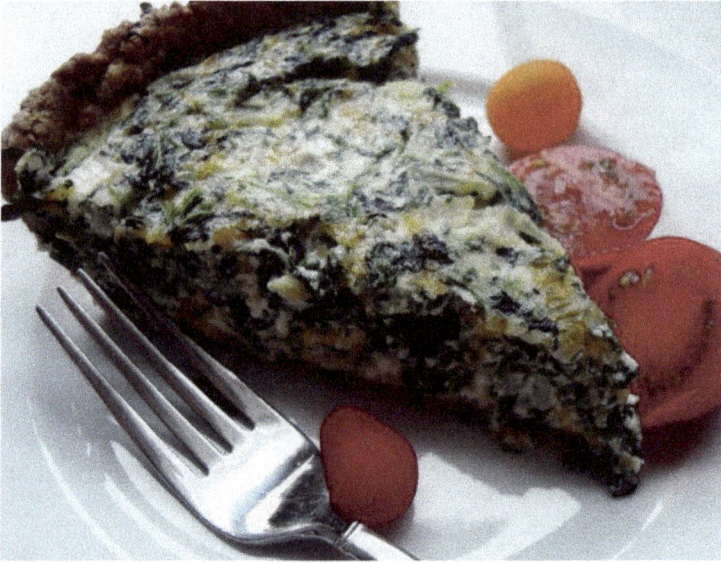

Servings: 4

Preparation Time: 10 minutes

Cooking Time: 4 hours

Ingredients:

- 10 ounces of frozen chopped spinach, thawed and squeezed
- 4 ounces of feta cheese, shredded
- 2 cups of unsweetened almond milk
- 4 eggs

- ¼ teaspoon of red pepper flakes, crushed
- Salt and ground black pepper, as required

Instructions:

1. In a baking dish, add all the ingredients and blend until well combined.
2. Arrange the baking dish over the wire rack.
3. Select "Slow Cooker" of Breville Smart Air Fryer Oven and assail "Low".
4. Set the timer for 4 hours and press "Start/Stop" to start cooking.
5. When the cooking time is completed, remove the baking dish from the oven and transfer the quiche onto a platter.
6. Cut into equal-sized wedges and serve hot.

Chicken & Spinach Quiche

Servings: 4

Preparation Time: 15 minutes

Cooking Time: 12 minutes

Ingredients:

- 2 ounces of cooked chicken, chopped
- ½ cup of fresh spinach, chopped
- ¼ cup of part-skim mozzarella cheese, shredded
- ½ cup of low-fat Parmesan cheese, shredded
- 2 tablespoons of unsweetened almond milk
- Salt and ground black pepper, as required

Instructions:

1. In a bowl, add all ingredients and blend well.
2. Transfer the mixture into a baking dish.
3. Select "Air Fry" of Breville Smart Air Fryer Oven and adjust the temperature to 320 degrees F.
4. Set the timer for 12 minutes and press "Start/Stop" to start preheating.

5. When the unit beeps to point out that it's preheated, arrange the baking dish over the wire rack.

6. When the cooking time is completed, remove the baking dish from oven and place onto a wire rack to chill for about 5 minutes before serving.

7. Cut into equal-sized wedges and serve hot.

Ground Chicken & Mushroom Frittata

Servings: 4

Preparation Time: 15 minutes

Cooking Time: 40 minutes

Ingredients:

- 2 tablespoons of olive oil, divided
- 8 ounces of ground chicken
- 8 ounces of fresh mushrooms, chopped
- 8 eggs
- 3 tablespoons of coconut cream
- 3 tablespoons of fresh parsley, chopped
- ¼ teaspoon of garlic powder
- Salt and ground black pepper, as required
- ½ cup of low-fat cheddar cheese, shredded

Instructions:

1. In a skillet, heat 1 tablespoon of oil over medium-high heat and cook the ground chicken for about 5 minutes, stirring frequently and ending the meat.
2. With a slotted spoon, place the cooked chicken into a bowl.

3. In the same skillet, heat the remaining tablespoon of oil over medium heat and cook the mushrooms for about 10 minutes, stirring occasionally.

4. Transfer the mushrooms into the bowl with cooked chicken and put aside to chill.

5. In a large bowl, add the eggs, coconut milk, parsley, thyme, onion powder, garlic powder, salt and black pepper and beat until well combined.

6. Add the cheese and stir to mix.

7. Add the chicken mixture and blend well.

8. Place the mixture into a greased baking pan.

9. Arrange the pan over the wire rack.

10. Select "Bake" of Breville Smart Air Fryer Oven and adjust the temperature to 325 degrees F.

11. Set the timer for 25 minutes and press "Start/Stop" to start preheating.

12. When the unit beeps to point out that it's preheated, insert the wire rack in the oven.

13. When the cooking time is completed, remove the pan from the oven and put aside to chill for five minutes before serving.

Salmon Quiche

Servings: 2

Preparation Time: 15 minutes

Cooking Time: 20 minutes

Ingredients:

- 5½ ounces of salmon fillet, chopped
- Salt and ground black pepper, as required
- ½ tablespoon of fresh lemon juice
- 1 egg yolk
- 3½ tablespoons of chilled coconut oil
- 2/3 cups of flour
- 1 tablespoon of cold water
- 2 eggs
- 3 tablespoons of whipping cream
- 1 scallion, chopped

Instructions:

1. In a bowl, add the salmon, salt, black pepper and juice and blend well.
2. In another bowl, add the ingredient, coconut oil, flour and water and blend until a dough forms.

3. Place the dough onto a floured smooth surface and roll into about 7-inch round.
4. Place the dough in a quiche pan and press firmly in the bottom and along the sides.
5. Trim the surplus edges.
6. In a small bowl, add the eggs, cream, salt and black pepper and beat until well combined.
7. Place the cream mixture over the crust evenly and top with the salmon mixture, followed by the scallion.
8. Select "Air Fry" of Breville Smart Air Fryer Oven and adjust the temperature to 355 degrees F.
9. Set the timer for 20 minutes and press "Start/Stop" to start preheating.
10. When the unit beeps to point out that it's preheated, arrange the quiche pan over the wire rack.
11. When the cooking time is completed, remove the quiche pan from the oven and put aside for about 5 minutes before serving.
12. Cut the quiche into equal-sized wedges and serve.

Beef & Mushroom Casserole

Servings: 6

Preparation Time: 15 minutes

Cooking Time: 19 minutes

Ingredients:

- 1 tablespoon of olive oil
- ½ pound ground beef
- ¾ cup of yellow onion, chopped
- 5 fresh mushrooms, sliced
- 8 eggs, beaten
- ½ teaspoon of garlic salt
- ¾ cup of low-fat Cheddar cheese, shredded and divided
- ¼ cup of sugar-free Alfredo sauce

Instructions:

1. In a skillet, heat the oil over medium heat and cook the meat and onions for about 4-5 minutes.
2. Add the mushrooms and cook for about 6-7 minutes.
3. Remove from the oven and drain the grease from the skillet.

4. In a bowl, add the meat mixture, beaten eggs, garlic salt, ½ cup of cheese and Alfredo sauce and stir to mix.

5. Place the meat mixture into a baking dish.

6. Select "Air Fry" of Breville Smart Air Fryer Oven and adjust the temperature to 390 degrees F.

7. Set the timer for 12 minutes and press "Start/Stop" to start preheating.

8. When the unit beeps to point out that it's preheated, arrange the baking dish over the wire rack.

9. After 6 minutes of cooking, stir the sausage mixture well.

10. When the cooking time is completed, remove the baking dish from oven and place onto a wire rack to chill for about 5 minutes before serving.

11. Cut into equal-sized wedges and serve with the topping of remaining cheese.

Chicken & Cauliflower Casserole

Servings: 5

Preparation Time: 15 minutes

Cooking Time: 35 minutes

Ingredients:

- 1½ tablespoons of olive oil
- ½ of large onion, chopped
- 24 ounces of cauliflower rice
- 3 eggs
- 2 tablespoons of unsweetened almond milk
- Salt and ground black pepper, as required
- ½ pound cooked chicken, chopped
- ¼ cup of low-fat Cheddar cheese, shredded

Instructions:

1. In a skillet, heat the oil over medium heat and sauté the onion for about 4-5 minutes.
2. Remove from the heat and transfer the onion into a bowl.
3. Add the cauliflower rice and blend well.
4. Place the mixture into a baking dish.

5. Select "Bake" of Breville Smart Air Fryer Oven and adjust the temperature to 350 degrees F.

6. Set the timer for 32 minutes and press "Start/Stop" to start preheating.

7. When the unit beeps to point out that it's preheated, arrange the baking dish over the wire rack.

8. Stir the mixture once after 8 minutes.

9. Meanwhile, in a bowl, add the eggs, milk, salt and black pepper and beat well.

10. After 15 minutes of cooking, place the egg mixture over cauliflower rice mixture evenly and top with the chicken pieces.

11. After 30 minutes of cooking, sprinkle the casserole with the cheese.

12. When the cooking time is completed, remove the baking dish from oven and place onto a wire rack to chill for about 5 minutes before serving.

13. Cut into equal-sized wedges and serve.

Eggs with Turkey & Spinach

Servings: 4

Preparation Time: 15 minutes

Cooking Time: 23 minutes

Ingredients:

- 1 tablespoon of coconut oil
- 1-pound fresh baby spinach
- 4 eggs
- 7 ounces of cooked turkey, chopped
- 4 teaspoons of unsweetened almond milk
- Salt and ground black pepper, as required

Instructions:

1. In a skillet, melt the coconut oil over medium heat and cook the spinach for about 2-3 minutes or until just wilted.
2. Remove from the heat and transfer the spinach into a bowl.
3. Put aside to chill slightly.
4. Divide the spinach into 4 greased ramekins, followed by the turkey.

5. Crack 1 egg into each ramekin and drizzle with almond milk.
6. Sprinkle with salt and black pepper.
7. Select "Air Fry" of Breville Smart Air Fryer Oven and adjust the temperature to 355 degrees F.
8. Set the timer for 20 minutes and press "Start/Stop" to start preheating.
9. When the unit beeps to point out that it's preheated, arrange the ramekins over the wire rack.
10. When the cooking time is completed, remove the ramekins from oven and place onto a wire rack to chill for about 5 minutes before serving.

Eggs with Turkey

Servings: 2

Preparation Time: 10 minutes

Cooking Time: 13 minutes

Ingredients:

- 2 teaspoons of coconut oil, softened
- 2 ounces of cooked turkey breast, sliced thinly
- 4 large eggs, divided
- 1 tablespoon of coconut milk
- Salt and ground black pepper, as required
- 1/8 teaspoon of smoked paprika
- 3 tablespoons of low-fat Parmesan cheese, grated finely
- 2 teaspoons of fresh chives, minced

Instructions:

1. In the bottom of a baking dish, spread the coconut oil.
2. Arrange the turkey slices over the coconut oil.
3. In a bowl, add 1egg, coconut milk, salt and black pepper and beat until smooth.
4. Place the egg mixture over the turkey slices evenly.

5. Carefully crack the remaining eggs on top and sprinkle with paprika, salt, black pepper, cheese and chives evenly.

6. Select "Air Fry" of Breville Smart Air Fryer Oven and adjust the temperature to 320 degrees F.

7. Set the timer for 13 minutes and press "Start/Stop" to start preheating.

8. When the unit beeps to point out that it's preheated, arrange the baking dish over the wire rack.

9. When the cooking time is completed, remove the baking dish from the oven and put aside for about 5 minutes before serving.

10. Cut into equal-sized wedges and serve.

Cranberry Muffins

Servings: 8

Preparation Time: 25 minutes

Cooking Time: 15 minutes

Ingredients:

- ¼ cup of unsweetened almond milk
- 2 large eggs
- ½ teaspoon of vanilla extract
- 1½ cups of almond flour
- ¼ cup of Erythritol
- 1 teaspoon of baking powder
- ¼ teaspoon of ground cinnamon
- 1/8 teaspoon of salt
- ½ cup of fresh cranberries
- ¼ cup of walnuts, chopped

Instructions:

1. In a blender, add the almond milk, eggs, vanilla, and pulse for about 20-30 seconds.

2. Add the almond flour, Erythritol, baking powder, cinnamon, salt, and pulse for about 30-45 seconds until well blended.
3. Transfer the mixture into a bowl.
4. Gently fold in half the cranberries and walnuts.
5. Place the mixture into 8 silicone muffin cups of and top each with remaining cranberries.
6. Select "Air Fry" of Breville Smart Air Fryer Oven and adjust the temperature to 325 degrees F.
7. Set the timer for 15 minutes and press "Start/Stop" to start preheating.
8. When the unit beeps to point out that it's preheated, arrange the muffin cups of over the wire rack.
9. When the cooking time is completed, remove the muffin cups of from oven and place onto a wire rack to chill for about 10 minutes.
10. Carefully invert the muffins onto the wire rack to completely cool before serving.

Savory Carrot Muffins

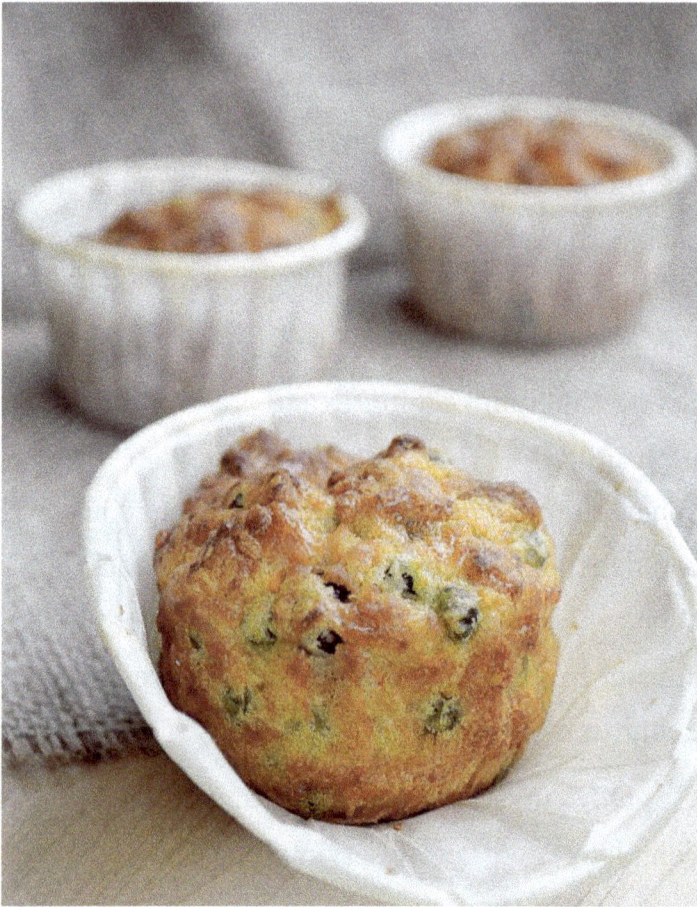

Servings: 6

Preparation Time: 15 minutes

Cooking Time: 7 minutes

Ingredients:

<u>For Muffins:</u>

- ¼ cup of whole-wheat flour
- ¼ cup of all-purpose flour
- ½ teaspoon of baking powder
- 1/8 teaspoon of baking soda
- ½ teaspoon of dried parsley, crushed
- ½ teaspoon of salt
- ½ cup of low-fat plain yoghurt
- 1 teaspoon of vinegar
- 1 tablespoon of olive oil
- 3 tablespoons of cottage cheese, grated
- 1 carrot, peeled and grated
- 2-4 tablespoons of water (if needed)

<u>For Topping:</u>

- 7 ounces of low-fat Parmesan cheese, grated
- ¼ cup of walnuts, chopped

Instructions:

1. For muffins: in a large bowl, mix together the flours, baking powder, baking soda, parsley, and salt.
2. In another large bowl, add the yoghurt and vinegar and blend well.

3. Add the remaining ingredients apart from water and beat them well. (Add some water if needed).
4. Make a well in the centre of the yoghurt mixture.
5. Slowly add the flour mixture in the well and blend until well combined.
6. Place the mixture into lightly greased 6 medium-sized muffin molds evenly and top with the Parmesan cheese and walnuts.
7. Select "Air Fry" of Breville Smart Air Fryer Oven and adjust the temperature to 355 degrees F.
8. Set the timer for 7 minutes and press "Start/Stop" to start preheating.
9. When the unit beeps to point out that it's preheated, arrange the muffin molds over the wire rack.
10. When the cooking time is completed, remove the muffin molds from the oven and place onto a wire rack to chill for about 5 minutes.
11. Carefully invert the muffins onto the platter and serve warm.

Chicken & Spinach Muffins

Servings: 6

Preparation Time: 10 minutes

Cooking Time: 17 minutes

Ingredients:

- 6 eggs
- ½ cup of unsweetened almond milk
- Salt and ground black pepper, as required
- 2 ounces of cooked chicken, chopped
- ¾ cup of fresh spinach, chopped

Instructions:

1. In a bowl, add the eggs, milk, salt and black pepper and beat until well combined.
2. Add the chicken and spinach and stir to mix.
3. Divide the spinach mixture into 6 greased cups of an egg bite mold evenly.
4. Select "Air Fry" of Breville Smart Air Fryer Oven and adjust the temperature to 325 degrees F.
5. Set the timer for 17 minutes and press "Start/Stop" to start preheating.

6. When the unit beeps to point out that it's preheated, arrange the egg bite mold over the wire rack.

7. When the cooking time is completed, remove the egg bite mold from oven and place onto a wire rack to chill for about 5 minutes.

8. Serve warm.

Zucchini Fritters

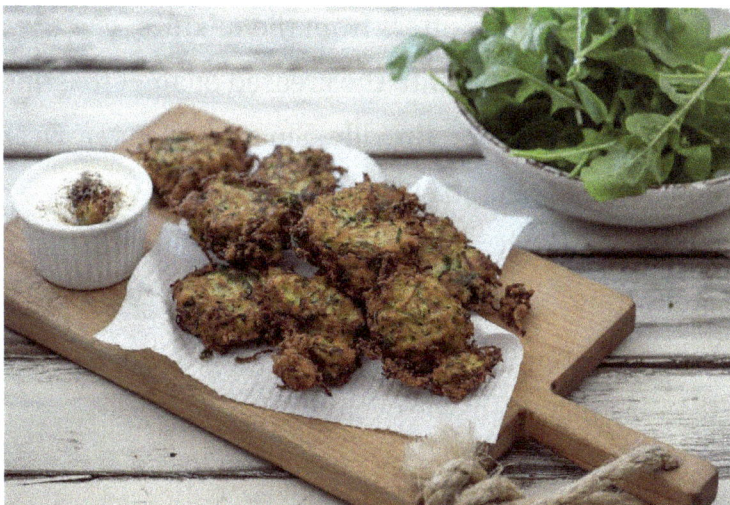

Servings: 4

Preparation Time: 15 minutes

Cooking Time: 7 minutes

Ingredients:

- 10½ ounces of zucchini, grated and squeezed
- 7 ounces of low-fat Halloumi cheese
- ¼ cup of almond flour
- 2 eggs
- 1 teaspoon of fresh dill, minced
- Salt and ground black pepper, as required

Instructions:

1. In a large bowl and blend together all the ingredients.
2. Make small-sized fritters from the mixture.
3. Arrange the fritters into the greased enamel roasting pan.
4. Select "Air Fry" of Breville Smart Air Fryer Oven and adjust the temperature to 355 degrees F.
5. Set the timer for 7 minutes and press "Start/Stop" to start preheating.
6. When the unit beeps to point out that it's preheated, insert the roasting pan in the oven.
7. When the cooking time is completed, remove the roasting pan from the oven.
8. Serve warm.

Onion Soup

Servings: 6

Preparation Time: 15 minutes

Cooking Time: 5 hours 10 minutes

Ingredients:

- 2 tablespoons of olive oil
- 2 medium sweet onions, sliced
- 2 garlic cloves, minced
- ¼ cup of low-sodium soy sauce
- 1 teaspoon of unsweetened applesauce
- 1 teaspoon of dried oregano, crushed
- 1 teaspoon of dried basil, crushed
- Ground black pepper, as required
- 5 cups of low-sodium vegetable broth
- ¼ cup of low-fat Parmesan cheese, grated

Instructions:

1. In an oven-safe pan that will put in the Breville Smart Air Fryer Oven, heat the oil over medium heat and cook the onion for about 8-9 minutes.
2. Add the garlic and cook for about 1 minute.

87

3. Remove from the heat and stir in the remaining ingredients apart from cheese.
4. Cover the pan with a lid.
5. Arrange the pan over the wire rack.
6. Select "Slow Cooker" of Breville Smart Air Fryer Oven and assail "Low".
7. Set the timer for five hours and press "Start/Stop" to start cooking.
8. When the cooking time is completed, remove the pan from the oven.
9. Remove the lid and stir in the cheese until melted completely.
10. Serve hot.

Mixed Veggies Soup

Servings: 6

Preparation Time: 15 minutes

Cooking Time: 8 hours 5 minutes

Ingredients:

- 1 tablespoon of olive oil
- 1 yellow onion, chopped
- 1 celery stalk, chopped
- 1 large carrot, peeled and chopped
- 2 garlic cloves, minced
- 1 teaspoon of dried oregano, crushed
- 1 large zucchini, chopped
- 2 tomatoes, chopped
- 1 cup of fresh spinach, chopped
- 4 cups of homemade low-sodium vegetable broth
- Salt and ground black pepper, as required

Instructions:

1. In an oven-safe pan that will put in the Breville Smart Air Fryer Oven, heat the oil over medium heat and sauté the onion, celery and carrot for about 3-4 minutes.

2. Add the garlic, thyme, and sauté for about 1 minute.

3. Remove from the heat and stir in the remaining ingredients.

4. Cover the pan with a lid.

5. Arrange the pan over the wire rack.

6. Select "Slow Cooker" of Breville Smart Air Fryer Oven and assail "Low".

7. Set the timer for 8 hours and press "Start/Stop" to start cooking.

8. When the cooking time is completed, remove the pan from the oven.

9. Remove the lid and stir the mixture well.

10. Serve hot.

Squash & Apple Soup

Servings: 6

Preparation Time: 15 minutes

Cooking Time: 8 hours

Ingredients:

- 5 cups of butternut squash, peeled and chopped
- 2 medium Granny Smith apples, peeled, cored and chopped
- 1 large carrot, peeled and chopped
- 1 small white onion, chopped
- 1 garlic clove, minced
- 4 cups of chicken broth
- 1 teaspoon of dried oregano, crushed
- 1 teaspoon of dried thyme, crushed
- Salt and ground black pepper, as required
- 1 cup of unsweetened coconut milk

Instructions:

1. In an oven-safe pan that will put in the Breville Smart Air Fryer Oven, add all ingredients apart from coconut milk and stir to mix.

2. Cover the pan with a lid.

3. Arrange the pan over the wire rack.

4. Select "Slow Cooker" of Breville Smart Air Fryer Oven and assail "High".

5. Set the timer for 8 hours and press "Start/Stop" to start cooking.

1. 6 After 4½ hours of cocking, stir in the coconut milk and cheese.

2. 7 When the cooking time is completed, remove the pan from the oven.

9. Open the lid and stir in the coconut milk.

10. With a stick blender, puree the soup until smooth.

11. Serve immediately.

Chicken & Spinach Soup

Servings: 6

Preparation Time: 15 minutes

Cooking Time: 6 hours

Ingredients:

- 2 tablespoons of coconut oil, melted
- 4 cups of cooked chicken, chopped
- 8 cups of fresh spinach, chopped
- 1 large carrot, peeled and chopped
- 1 small onion, chopped finely
- ½ tablespoon of garlic, minced
- Salt and ground black pepper, as required
- 6 cups of low-sodium chicken broth

Instructions:

1. In an oven-safe pan that will put in the Breville Smart Air Fryer Oven, place all ingredients and stir to mix.
2. Cover the pan with a lid.
3. Arrange the pan over the wire rack.

4. Select "Slow Cooker" of Breville Smart Air Fryer Oven and assail "Low".

5. Set the timer for six hours and press "Start/Stop" to start cooking.

6. When the cooking time is completed, remove the pan from the oven.

7. Remove the lid and serve hot.

Chicken & Carrot Stew

Servings: 6

Preparation Time: 15 minutes

Cooking Time: 6 hours

Ingredients:

- 4 (5-ounce of) boneless chicken breast, cubed
- 3 cups of carrots, peeled and cubed
- 2 celery stalks, chopped
- 1 medium yellow onion, chopped
- 2 garlic cloves, minced
- Salt and ground black pepper, as required
- ½ teaspoon of dried thyme
- ½ teaspoon of dried rosemary
- 2 cups of chicken broth
- 2 tablespoons of olive oil

Instructions:

1. In an oven-safe pan that will put in the Breville Smart Air Fryer Oven, place all ingredients apart from oil and stir to mix.
2. Cover the pan with a lid.

3. Arrange the pan over the wire rack.

4. Select "Slow Cooker" of Breville Smart Air Fryer Oven and assail "Low".

5. Set the timer for six hours and press "Start/Stop" to start cooking.

6. When the cooking time is completed, remove the pan from the oven and serve hot.

7. Open the lid and stir in the oil.

8. Serve hot.

Turkey Meatballs & Spinach Soup

Servings: 6

Preparation Time: 20 minutes

Cooking Time: 6 hours 5 minutes

Ingredients:

For Meatballs:

- 2 pounds lean ground turkey
- 4 garlic cloves, minced
- ¼ cup of fresh cilantro, chopped
- 1 egg
- 2 teaspoons of dried rosemary, crushed
- Salt and ground black pepper, as required
- 2 tablespoons of olive oil

For Soup:

- 1 carrot, peeled and sliced large
- 1 large tomato, chopped
- 1 celery stalk, chopped
- 1 small onion, chopped
- Salt and ground black pepper, as required
- 7 cups of low-sodium chicken broth

- 6 cups of fresh spinach, chopped

Instructions:

1. For meatballs: in a large bowl, add all the ingredients apart from oil and blend until well combined.
2. Make small sized balls from the mixture.
3. In a skillet, heat the oil over medium heat and cook the meatballs for about 4-5 minutes or until golden brown from all sides.
1. 4 With a slotted spoon, transfer the meatballs onto a plate.
2. 5 In an oven-safe pan that will put in the Breville Smart Air Fryer Oven, place the celery, onion, carrot and tomato.
6. Place the meatballs over the veggies.
7. Cover the pan with a lid.
8. Arrange the pan over the wire rack.
9. Select "Slow Cooker" of Breville Smart Air Fryer Oven and assail "Low".
10. Set the timer for six hours and press "Start/Stop" to start cooking.
11. When the cooking time is completed, remove the pan from the oven and immediately, stir in the spinach.
12. Cover the pan with a lid for about 5 minutes before serving.

Cheesy Beef Soup

Servings: 8

Preparation Time: 15 minutes

Cooking Time: 5½ hours

Ingredients:

- 3 tablespoons of coconut oil
- 1 medium onion, chopped
- 2 celery stalks, chopped
- 2 large cloves garlic, minced
- 1-pound cooked beef, chopped
- 5 cups of low-sodium beef broth
- Salt and ground black pepper, as required
- 1 cup of full-fat coconut milk
- 1½ cups of low-fat Swiss cheese, shredded

Instructions:

1. In an oven-safe pan that will put in the Breville Smart Air Fryer Oven, melt the butter over medium heat and sauté the onion, celery and garlic and cook for about 5 minutes.
2. Stir in the beef, broth, salt and black pepper and take away from the heat.

99

3. Cover the pan with a lid.

4. Arrange the pan over the wire rack.

5. Select "Slow Cooker" of Breville Smart Air Fryer Oven and assail "High".

6. Set the timer for 5½ hours and press "Start/Stop" to start cooking.

7. After 4½ hours of cocking, stir in the coconut milk and cheese.

8. When the cooking time is completed, remove the pan from the oven.

9. Open the lid and serve hot.

Beef Meatballs & Zucchini Soup

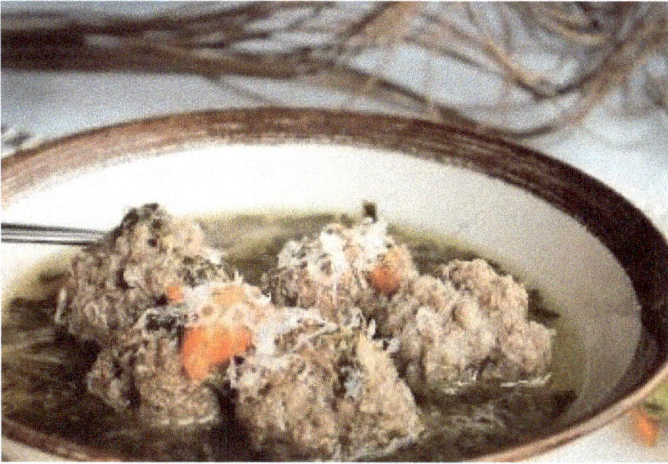

Servings: 8

Preparation Time: 20 minutes

Cooking Time: 6 hours 10 minutes

Ingredients:

For Meatballs:

- 2 pounds lean ground beef
- 4 garlic cloves, minced
- ¼ cup of fresh parsley leaves, chopped
- ½ cup of Parmesan cheese, grated
- 1 egg, beaten

- 1 teaspoon of dried oregano, crushed
- 1 teaspoon of dried rosemary, crushed
- Salt and ground black pepper, as required
- 2 tablespoons of coconut oil

For Soup:

- 1 celery stalk, chopped
- 1 small onion, chopped
- 1 small carrot, peeled and chopped
- 1 large plum tomato, chopped finely
- 3 large zucchinis, spiralized with a blade
- Salt and ground black pepper, as required
- 8 cups of low-sodium beef broth

Instructions:

1. For meatballs in a large bowl, add all ingredients and blend until well combined.
2. Make small sized balls from the mixture.
3. In a large skillet, heat the oil over medium heat and cook the meatballs for about 4-5 minutes or until golden brown from all sides.
4. With a slotted spoon, transfer the meatballs onto a plate.
5. In an oven-safe pan that will put in the Breville Smart Air Fryer Oven, place the celery, onion, carrot and tomato.

6. Place the zucchini noodles over vegetables and sprinkle with salt and black pepper.

7. Place the broth over vegetables.

8. Carefully add meatballs in broth mixture.

9. Cover the pan with a lid.

10. Arrange the pan over the wire rack.

11. Select "Slow Cooker" of Breville Smart Air Fryer Oven and assail "Low".

12. Set the timer for six hours and press "Start/Stop" to start cooking.

13. When the cooking time is completed, remove the pan from the oven and serve hot.

Ground Beef & Veggies Soup

Servings: 6

Preparation Time: 15 minutes

Cooking Time: 8¼ hours

Ingredients:

- 1 tablespoon of olive oil
- 1 yellow onion, chopped
- 2 garlic cloves, minced
- 1 teaspoon of dried oregano, crushed
- 1½ pounds ground beef
- 2 tomatoes, chopped
- 1 large zucchini, chopped
- 1 cup of fresh kale, tough ribs removed and chopped
- 5 cups of vegetable broth
- Salt and ground black pepper, as required

Instructions:

1. In an oven-safe pan that will put in the Breville Smart Air Fryer Oven, heat the oil over medium heat and sauté the onion for about 3-4 minutes.
2. Add the garlic and thyme and sauté for about 1 minute.

3. Add the meat and cook for about 4-5 minutes.

4. Add the tomatoes and cook for about 4-5 minutes.

5. Remove from the heat and stir in the remaining ingredients.

6. Cover the pan with a lid.

7. Arrange the pan over the wire rack.

8. Select "Slow Cooker" of Breville Smart Air Fryer Oven and assail "Low".

9. Set the timer for 8 hours and press "Start/Stop" to start cooking.

10. When the cooking time is completed, remove the pan from the oven.

11. Remove the lid and stir the mixture well.

12. Serve hot.

Beef & Cabbage Stew

Servings: 8

Preparation Time: 15 minutes

Cooking Time: 9 hours

Ingredients:

- 2 pounds beef stew meat, trimmed and cubed
- Salt and ground black pepper, as required
- 5 cups of green cabbage, chopped
- 1 large onion, chopped
- 6 garlic cloves, minced
- 4 medium fresh tomatoes, chopped
- 1 cup of beef broth
- 2 tablespoons of fresh parsley, chopped

Instructions:

1. In an oven-safe pan that will put in the Breville Smart Air Fryer Oven, place all ingredients apart from parsley and stir to mix.
2. Cover the pan with a lid.
3. Arrange the pan over the wire rack.

4. Select "Slow Cooker" of Breville Smart Air Fryer Oven and assail "Low".

5. Set the timer for 9 hours and press "Start/Stop" to start cooking.

6. When the cooking time is completed, remove the pan from the oven and serve hot.

7. Open the lid and serve hot with the garnishing of parsley.

Beef & Mushroom Stew

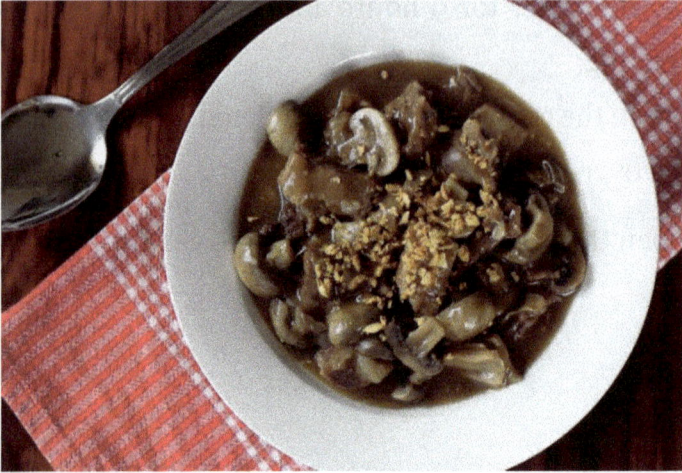

Servings: 8

Preparation Time: 15 minutes

Cooking Time: 8 hours

Ingredients:

- 2 pounds beef stew meat, cubed
- 2 cups of fresh mushrooms, sliced
- 4 garlic cloves, minced
- 1 cup of fresh parsley leaves, chopped
- 2 cups of tomato paste
- 2 cups of beef broth

- Salt and ground black pepper, as required

Instructions:

1. In an oven-safe pan that will put in the Breville Smart Air Fryer Oven, place all ingredients and stir to mix.
2. Cover the pan with a lid.
3. Arrange the pan over the wire rack.
4. Select "Slow Cooker" of Breville Smart Air Fryer Oven and assail "Low".
5. Set the timer for 8 hours and press "Start/Stop" to start cooking.
6. When the cooking time is completed, remove the pan from the oven and serve hot.
7. Open the lid and serve hot.

www.ingramcontent.com/pod-product-compliance
Lightning Source LLC
Chambersburg PA
CBHW050754030426
42336CB00012B/1806